# Intermittent Fasting Playbook

*Your Ultimate Guide To Weight Loss, Burning Fat, Healing Your Body and Living a Healthy Lifestyle*

**Nicholas Mayor**

# Table of Contents

# Introduction

The global weight loss industry is a multi-billion dollar annual industry. To be precise, it was worth $168 billion in 2016 and is projected to reach between $278 billion and $442 billion by 2025. That's billions with a capital B. We're talking big money. The market is definitely huge.

Unfortunately, there is a dark side to all of this. There is a big reason why this market is so huge. Failure is the sad reality behind these numbers.

Every single year, people make New Year's resolutions to lose weight and they do the following. It's all too predictable. In fact, people from all four corners of the globe go through this same pattern. It happens without fail.

First, they get all excited about buying diet supplements. They would buy one supplement after another. They would also sign up for gym memberships. Some people would buy exercise equipment after seeing great videos on YouTube,

Facebook as well as dedicated cable shopping networks. Finally, a large number of people would buy one diet book after another.

Right when they start, they see some results. Again, this happens pretty much across the board. This doesn't happen to everybody, but this happens, generally speaking.

They lose a few pounds here and there. In fact, a lot of these people start developing a leaner and more muscular frame. Things look like their weight loss plans are panning out.

Unfortunately, it also follows that, sooner or later, the fat returns. That's right. They end up dumping the diet book, they stop going to the gym, they switch supplements or stop taking supplements altogether, and they end up where they began.

The problem? Most weight loss programs are simply not sustainable. These people go back to their old eating lifestyle habits. It is no surprise that the weight keeps coming back. In fact, in many cases, they end up in a worse place.

How? They just get bigger and bigger. That's right. Not only did the few pounds that you lost on your diet come back, but you actually made certain changes to your system that made it so much easier to pack on more pounds. You end up in a worse place.

If any of this applies to you, I've got good news for you. If you are in any way, shape or form sick and tired of failing with your diet, this book can be the last weight loss book you will ever need. Seriously. Real story. See you in Chapter 1.

# Chapter 1: How Real Weight Loss Works

If you think about it hard enough, weight loss is not rocket science. Far from it. It's actually a simple mathematical equation: eat less, move around more. I know that sounds pretty basic, but that's really all there is to it.

There is a third option, but most people have a tough time with this third option. The third options, of course, is to do both.

But the bottom line is, if you want to lose weight and finally get rid of that nasty looking spare tire around your midsection, you just need to do one or both of these things: eat less, move around more.

When you eat less, you reduce the amount of calories you take in every single day.

Calories are crucial for your body to keep body and soul together. Your body uses calories as fuel. Without calories coming in, your body starts to look for a replacement source of energy. This is where the weight loss comes in.

For example, if you normally take in 1,500 calories every day and you drop that down to 700 or even 500, what do you think happens? That's right, your body would start burning muscle or fat to make up for the calorie shortfall.

In fact, if you keep this up long enough, your body will burn through that thick layer of fat all over your body, from your fat cheeks to your fat neck, to the flabby handles around your midsection, to the drooping fatty curtains at the bottom of your arms, or the fat layers at the back of your thighs and around your hips that look like cottage cheese.

Regardless of whatever fat layers your body has managed to accumulate over the years, you can burn through these by simply cutting down on the amount of calories you eat every single day.

You can also take the opposite approach. You can choose to move around more. In other words, you can eat the same amount of food, but choose to exercise or engage in higher levels of physical activity.

I can't emphasize the latter part enough. A lot of people are under the impression that moving around more simply means hitting the gym. They think that they have to get a bike or start swimming. It doesn't have to involve any of that. Seriously.

In fact, you can just do whatever you're doing now and just increase your daily activity. Maybe you walk a certain number of feet to get to work, maybe you take the stairs from time to time, or maybe you lift certain things at work. By increasing your amount of daily activity, you just increase the intensity as well as the duration of these activities.

For example, instead of always parking very close to the entrance of the mall, your office, or any other building you go to on a regular basis, make it a practice to park as far away as possible. I understand that this is inconvenient. This is definitely not all that comfortable, but you'll get used to it.

When you do that, you incorporate into your daily physical routine increased activity. Believe it or not, parking several hundred feet away from the entrance can burn a lot more calories than if you had parked right in front of the entrance.

The same logic applies to your use of the elevator. Believe me, the elevator is one amazing modern convenience. Most of us cannot live without an elevator. But if you were to make it a habit to walk a few stories every single day and then take the elevator for the rest of your trip, this can help you lose a lot of weight.

Please understand that when it comes to increasing your daily amount of physical activity, the secret is consistency. You're not doing yourself any favors if you run a lot or sweat a lot or otherwise push yourself physically for one day of the week and then go back to your old routine for the rest of the week. That's just not going to work. That's not going to cut it.

You have to engage in an increased level of physical activity even though it's a marginal improvement on a day to day basis. This means that you don't have to be a hero. You don't have to go overboard. You don't have to overdo it.

For example, if you normally walk 150 steps every single day, you can ramp it up to 175 and lose a lot of weight. How? Well, if you can stick to that physical activity level day after day, week after week, month after month, you will see profound changes.

Again, the key here is consistency. A little bit of consistency goes a long way.

As powerful as this advice may be, and this is a proven scientific fact, there is a problem. Seriously. There is a problem with this weight loss equation. It doesn't really matter whether you're trying to cut down on the calories you eat or increase the amount of physical activity you do every single day. There is one wall that you will keep hitting.

Why? Well, here's the thing. All weight loss programs and systems are variations of the principles above.

That's right. From the most fancy, highfalutin food supplement to the most amazing looking workout equipment, or even the most exclusive gym membership, they all go back to that weight loss equation. Either you eat less or you move around more.

Ideally, you should do both. But if you were to break down and analyze all these different weight loss programs, products and systems available on the market, they all come back to those two principles. Either they focus on appetite suppression or calorie burning.

Sounds good so far, right? Well, here's the problem. All these solutions leave out one crucial ingredient. This is the ingredient that will make or break your weight loss success.

What is the ingredient? Discipline. Seriously. Discipline.

If you were to stick to a program and choose to be consistent, persistent and persevere despite the pain, the inconvenience, the discomfort, you will get fit. You will lose all that flab. You will start looking better. Your self esteem would improve. You would become more confident.

Unfortunately, almost all the weight loss systems out there leave this out. They get you all pumped up about the machine. They get you all excited about the "revolutionary" new way you can cut down on calories. This is all well and good, but without this crucial ingredient of discipline and the routine that it brings to the table, failure is only around the corner. It may take a long time.

I remember I lost 50 pounds and it took me about 8 years to get all that weight back, and then some. Without consistency and routine, whatever weight you manage to lose will come back. It's only a matter of time. It will happen sooner or later.

This is why it's really important to stop thinking about weight loss in terms of gimmicks, techniques, products or systems. Get those concepts out of your mind. Instead, focus on the missing ingredient. Again, it's all about discipline and routine.

Whatever weight loss method you choose must be consistent, persistent and become part of your daily routine. In fact, I would take things a step further. Your weight loss program must become part of who you are as a person.

As you can probably tell, most people fail to do this. In fact, most people do not even recognize the importance of discipline and routine in their efforts to lose weight. It is no surprise that most people just jump from one diet to another, one supplement to another, one gym membership to another, and one exercise machine to another.

It's as if they are on a carousel. They go round and round. They switch horses, but they end up in the same place. They're just going around. They're just chasing their tail.

You have to understand that your weight loss is very simple. In fact, you just need to move around and you will lose weight.

In a 2016 study by Professor Herman Pontzer of City University of New York, physical movement is important for health. It helps you become healthier overall.

Similarly, if you choose to cut down on calorie intake or you switch to higher quality calories, you can lose weight. In fact, it can make you healthier overall.

In a 2004 study out of Harvard, researcher Matthias B. Schulze showed that when people increase the amount of sugary or sweet drinks they consume, the fatter they got. They also increased their disease risks.

Finally, in a study out of the University of Otago in Wellington, New Zealand, a team of researchers led by Dr. Wright published in 2017 a study that indicates high green vegetable diets improves health outcomes. Not only does this type of diet increase weight loss, but it also reduces the risk of a range of chronic diseases.

# Chapter 2: The Real Reason Why People Fail to Lose Weight and Keep It Off

I wish I could tell you that the reason why most people fail to lose weight is because of something outside of them. I wish it was some sort of external circumstance or some sort of factor beyond their control. The problem, however, strikes closer to home. The problem is lack of discipline.

This is going to be a major hurdle because, last time I checked, you can't pack discipline into a capsule. You really can't. There is no tablet that you can buy from a store that makes you more disciplined, focused and persistent. There is no pharmaceutical product that reforms your mental and physical system to such an extent that you adopt a new routine that helps you lose weight.

The sad reality is that you cannot break your lifestyle habits overnight. They become part of you. In fact, discipline plays such a big role in weight loss that it really goes a long way in ensuring success or bringing on failure.

In a 2007 study out of the University of Sheffield, researcher Myles Balfe showed that discipline and dieting are tightly linked. In his study of young adults with Type I diabetes, study subjects who had a tough time maintaining discipline as far as their diet and exercise routines go, actually got worse over time. This indicates the strong link between discipline and lifestyle.

Lifestyle, of course, involves moving around as well as eating. We're not just talking about random calories here. We're also talking about food choices.

This might seem pretty straightforward, but here's the problem. You can't just slip on a new routine. You can't just say to yourself that since you need to lose weight that you are going to automatically choose to do things differently. It just doesn't work that way.

It all goes back to the fact that you cannot break your habits overnight. It took some time for you to adopt those habits, whether you liked them or not, and it's going to take some time for you to lose them.

Interestingly enough, we choose our habits. I know it will shock a lot of people because, hey, let's face it, all of us have at least one bad habit.

How can I say that you chose your bad habits? Well, think about it, for you to repeat a behavior, you have to have some sort of reward. It's what keeps you coming back. This reward is the incentive that pushes you to engage in that behavior over and over again.

This is chosen. This is not something that somebody imposed on you. It's not like somebody pointed a gun at you and said, "You're going to feel really good after eating that slice of chocolate cake" or "Your self esteem is going to improve after you chill out and play video games instead of hitting the gym." These are choices.

The deliberation process may be lightning quick. We may not even be aware of them, but we still chose them. And, initially, we're more conscious of the choice, but as time goes by and the more we repeat these behaviors, the more automatic everything seems to become. Again, you cannot break your habits overnight.

## Your Eating Lifestyle Needs to Change

Unfortunately, for things to turn around as far as your weight goes, your eating lifestyle needs to change. I'm not just talking about you eating a lot of food. I'm talking about your eating lifestyle.

In other words, your relationship to food, your mindset, and your routine regarding food. If this doesn't change, you're going to be stuck with the familiar pattern I described at the beginning of this book.

When you adopt a new diet, you lose a few pounds here and there. Things look really good at the outset. It seems that you have achieved some sort of breakthrough. In many cases, a lot of people finally lost pounds that they thought they would never ever pull off.

But unfortunately, all that weight keeps coming back. This is due to the fact that they did not change their eating lifestyle. They changed what they chose to eat. I mean, a lot of fad diets require that you eat certain foods and you skip others.

That's not the problem. The problem is not picking out certain types of food to eat. The problem is your relationship to food. That's where the struggle comes from.

The challenge is rooted in your attitude towards eating. This is the key to losing weight and keeping that weight off.

The problem, unfortunately, with most weight loss programs is that they focus on you taking stuff off your plate. Again, it's all about choosing to eat certain foods and not others. You feel that someone, somewhere, somehow, is imposing on you.

At the other side of the weight loss equation, the same thing applies. Maybe you read a book about rapid belly fat burning exercises. It lists all sorts of exercises you should do. Well, your mind still interprets this as somebody imposing new workouts or activities on you. After all, this is not really the kind of stuff that you normally do.

What is the net effect of all of this? Well, your body and mind will resist. It doesn't get any simpler than that. Your body and mind will put up a fight.

It may not be obvious, but sooner or later, you find yourself bargaining with yourself. You're saying to yourself, "Well, I normally wake up at 4 AM because I know that this jump starts my day and I am more likely to put in a good workout. I'm more likely to run a farther distance and I'm more likely to sweat a lot."

But it's raining outside or there's a mild drizzle. You come up with all sorts of excuses to not do it.

And sooner or later, the cheat day becomes a cheat week. The cheat week becomes a cheat month. And before you know it, you're back to doing what you normally do. You're back to your overweight habits.

What if I told you that there is a better way? Instead of taking stuff off your plate or feeling like you're being imposed upon, why not just reschedule and displace?

## Reschedule with Intermittent Fasting

Intermittent fasting is a weight loss system that pays more attention to when you eat instead of what you eat. Instead of obsessing about the things that you put in your mouth, intermittent fasting turns your attention to when you choose to eat.

Believe it or not, by simply scheduling your meals the right way, you end up losing weight. It seems almost effortless at a certain point. It becomes part of your routine. It becomes part of your eating lifestyle.

It doesn't seem like it's imposed by somebody out there. It doesn't seem like you're doing something out of the ordinary. Instead, you feel that intermittent fasting is just part of how you do things.

This is how you get out from under the discipline and routine requirements of long term or permanent weight loss. That's how you make progress. It's all about scheduling.

The second prong of this long term weight loss system is displacement. Instead of obsessing about taking stuff off your plate or avoiding certain foods, add foods to your plate.

But just like with any example of water displacement in real life, a lot of the stuff that you previously had will be pushed out of the way because you have added new foods to your weight loss lifestyle.

This is how displacement works. You're not just going to displace with any kind of random food. Instead, you're going to displace with calorie packed, high fat, low carb food. This is how you get faster and more sustainable results.

In the following chapters, I'm going to walk you through intermittent fasting, how it operates, its definition, and how you can implement it in your daily life.

# Chapter 3: What IF Is and Isn't

Usually, when people hear or read the word "fasting", they get scared. I really can't say I blame them. I mean last time I checked going for long extended periods of time without eating is quite inconvenient, if not downright uncomfortable, for most people.

This is why there are a lot of misconceptions regarding intermittent fasting. After all, it does have the word "fasting" in it. What if I told you that intermittent fasting is not actual fasting? You would probably sit up and pay attention, right? You probably would be less scared of this particular lifestyle protocol.

The truth is intermittent fasting is not actual fasting. Regardless of the label, you still eat within a twenty-four-hour period. The big difference is when you eat within that twenty-four-hour period. This is precisely the point behind intermittent fasting. When you eat is as important as what you choose to eat.

The vast majority of diets and weight-loss systems out there focus on eating certain foods and ignoring certain classes of foods. That's how they normally lay out their diet guidelines.

Unfortunately, as I mentioned in a previous chapter, most of them fail. Regardless of how much weight you lose initially, eventually all that weight will come back.

Intermittent fasting is different. It works with your body clock to increase the likelihood of you adopting a new routine. As I've mentioned in the previous chapter, this routine adoption is actually the key to sustainable weight loss.

It's not identifying a certain class of food. It definitely has nothing to do with the supplement you choose. This also has nothing to do with exercise machines. If you want to stick to a certain routine and continue to benefit from it for a long time to come, you must have some sort of mechanism.

Unfortunately, the vast majority of weight-loss systems, programs, diet books, supplements and other products available on the market are simply not up to the job. They're simply not sustainable.

Intermittent fasting just works with what you already do. Obviously, you eat every single day. It doesn't change that. What it changes is the window of time in which you eat.

## Intermittent Fasting and Confusing Intermittent Fasting "Flavors"

If you have done any kind of research on intermittent fasting, you probably have come up with different "protocols" or "flavors" of intermittent fasting. There are quite a number of them available on the Internet.

Unfortunately, the more of these you find, the easier it is to get confused. A lot of people are under the impression that intermittent fasting is the same as Eat

Stop Eat, The Warrior Diet, so on and so forth. They're different from each other.

You have to understand that intermittent fasting in of itself is a specific system. There are certain components or certain practices that define intermittent fasting. This can all be boiled down to simply watching the window of time in which you eat.

You eat within a twenty-four-hour period. You're still eating on a day-to-day basis. The only thing you changed, and this is the big deal behind IF, is when you choose to eat within that twenty-four-hour window.

Defined in these terms, intermittent fasting is different from Eat Stop Eat. As you can tell by the name of that protocol, you actually stop eating. You go on a regular day of eating and then you stop for a whole day then you start again. That requires actual fasting.

Fasting is defined as going on a twenty-four-hour period of no eating. Maybe you're drinking liquids. Perhaps you're drinking certain shakes but you're not eating solid food.

Similarly, intermittent fasting is not The Warrior Diet. The Warrior Diet uses eating scheduling where you stop eating. There is a period of time where you completely shut off all food-based calories. That isn't intermittent fasting.

Another common misconception regarding IF involves starvation. A lot of people are convinced that it is some sort of starvation diet. It isn't. How can it? You're still eating within a twenty-four-hour period. In fact, if you think about how it works and why it works, it isn't a diet at all.

Again, diets are all about calorie suppression. They're all about reducing the amount of calories you eat in any given day so your body can burn more calories than it takes in.

As you have learned from the initial chapter to this book, when you do that, you achieve a negative calorie state. Your body then starts burning fat or muscle mass to make up for the "lost" calories. That's how you lose weight.

That's how most diets work. It's all about calorie suppression. Maybe they would mix in a little increased activity or they would increase your body's natural passive metabolism. Still, regardless of the different modifications, it all goes back to the same formula: reducing calorie intake.

Defined in those terms, intermittent fasting is not a diet at all. You can still eat the same yummy food that you have always enjoyed. You can still eat the same amount of food. You just have to watch the time.

## Why Adopt Intermittent Fasting?

As I mentioned in a previous chapter to this book, the main reason most diets fail is the fact that your routine doesn't change. Sooner or later, you go back to your old routine. Discipline is crucial to sustainable weight loss.

Unfortunately, you cannot buy discipline in a capsule. It doesn't ship in a tablet. It's something that you have to work on day after day. It's something that you only manage to achieve when you overcome temptation and procrastination.

It is no surprise that people, especially in the United States, have a tough time establishing self-discipline. We live in a society where we're supposed to have our cake and eat too. In fact, we live in a society where it's perfectly okay and even expected that people should have dessert before their main meal. That's what you're going up against. It is no surprise that diets fail within this context because your mindset simply is not prepared.

With intermittent fasting, you work with your existing preferences. You're not really changing much except for one element: timing. You're still eating every single day. You're still enjoying the same foods that you have liked before.

Compare this to the typical diet where you basically shift to a whole new set of food or you add certain supplements to your daily meal plan. Instead, you just shift eating to a certain time frame within the day.

You also have a choice. It's not like there is some sort of one-size-fits-all formula. You can do it in one of two ways. It's not like you're imposing a totally alien or foreign system on yourself.

Finally, intermittent fasting works because it doesn't shock your system. As I have mentioned in a previous chapter, your number one enemy, as far as long-lasting personal changes are concerned, is yourself.

Let's face it human beings are creatures of habit. We grow accustomed to doing things a certain way. We grow accustomed to eating a certain way. It's very hard to break these patterns.

This is why when you adopt a hot, new diet fad, you are able to lose initially. This happens because you shocked your system into changing but, eventually, your body and mind rebel. It's not going to be obvious but, eventually, it creeps up on you. Sooner or later, you go back to your old patterns.

The reason for this, of course, is the fact that your new food lifestyle is just too much of a break from your previous lifestyle. Let's face it most diets really boil down to stopping eating. Either you stop eating altogether or you stop eating certain foods. This is too much. It shocks your system and guess what? Your system will push back. It's only a matter of time.

**Intermittent Fasting is Not the Final Destination to Weight Loss**

Another common misconception of regarding intermittent fasting is that it is the one-size-fits-all or final destination for personal weight loss. It isn't. The truth is it gives you a starting point. It gives you a routine. Once you get accustomed to it, you can choose to scale things up for better results.

Let me tell you the moment you drastically cut back on the calories you eat on a sustainable level is the moment you will finally get to say goodbye to all that fat. The open issue here is how to get there.

The great thing about intermittent fasting is that it helps you step start the process fairly rapidly. Once you've gotten used to it, you can scale up. There are actually many ways to do it, but here are the two most common ways for it.

First, you can scale up to Eat Stop Eat. I've mentioned this above. Eat Stop Eat, of course, means there is a period of time where you're eating and then there's a period of days where you just stop eating then you resume eating again.

Maybe you would stop for one day and then go back to eating for two days and then go back to one day of fasting. Whatever the case may be you scale up by experiencing a full twenty-four-hour period of no eating. That is Eat Stop Eat.

In fact, if you get good at it and you get used to it, you can adopt a 2-2-2 schedule. You can go two days of eating then two days of fasting then back to eating and so on and so forth.

Alternatively, you can scale up to 3-4-3. This is the second most common option. You go three days of eating and then four days of no food and then three days of eating, so one and so forth.

Sounds exciting, right? When you reach that stage, you are burning up a tremendous amount of calories assuming you keep up your daily activities. In other words, in the weight loss equation, everything remains the same as far as the metabolism and daily physical activity section is concerned. You just reduce calorie intake on the other end of the equation.

To reach this stage, you have to focus on your mindset and you have to build up discipline. These are really the main benefits you get with the intermittent fasting system. You can finally get out from under the very frustrating lose-gain-lose pattern that you get with most diets and weight loss systems. Intermittent fasting can supply the missing ingredients of discipline and routine that are sorely lacking with other methods of weight loss.

I wish I could tell you that this is easy. I wish I could tell you that this is something that you just adopt and things go swimmingly well. It doesn't work that way. It takes work.

Any time you change the things that you normally do, you're going to come up against your old habits. You're going to have to confront and deal with your old behavioral patterns. Oftentimes, these are hard to shake off. As I mentioned above, we do grow accustomed to doing things a certain way.

The good news is if you keep this up for long enough, the power of habit kicks in. There's an old saying that if you stick to a routine for twenty-one days, it becomes a habit. It becomes really hard for you to shake it off. That idea has undergone quite a bit of criticism. Some researchers are saying that the actual figure is closer to sixty days.

Regardless of whether you adopt or break a habit in twenty-one days or sixty days doesn't matter. What matters is that you stick to it long enough until it becomes a part of your routine.

# Chapter 4: Take This to Heart before You Begin

At this point, you're probably all excited about starting your journey into intermittent fasting. I can't say I blame you. It is exciting stuff because, after all, it has a lot going for it. It is not a diet. It is not some sort of exercise routine. Instead, it's just a simple modification to your daily schedule.

It seems so simple, so cut and dried, and so basic. You're probably very eager to try it out right here right now.

Well, before you jump in with both feet, please understand that you have to do some preliminary thinking first. You have to make sure that your mind is in the right place. You have to take to heart the following lessons; otherwise, your intermittent fasting journey is probably not going to end well.

I don't mean to be a joy-kill, but this is the truth. How many diets have you gotten excited about in the past? How many of them have succeeded? Well, let's put it this way. If they succeeded, then you wouldn't be reading this book, right?

Now that I have your attention, please pay attention to the following. In a 2014 study conducted by the Department of Health's Health Promotion unit out of the Public Health Foundation of India, Himanshu Gupta and associates showed that self-motivation and commitment to weight loss are crucial to long-term weight loss.

In their article in the International Journal of Preventive Medicine, they showed a link between one's ability to motivate oneself and commit to a certain course of action and long-term weight loss. In other words, these researchers identified key ingredients to long-term weight loss. You can lose weight easily with all sorts of fad diets out there. They're a dime a dozen. That's not the issue.

The issue is keeping that way off. This is where self-motivation and commitment come in. Unless you pay attention to what I'm about to say, it's going to be very hard for you to stick to the program. Regardless of how excited you are, it's only a matter of time until you get off the program. You can take that to the bank. That's guaranteed.

This is why you have to get your mind right. Your mind must be in the right place. You have to prepare yourself mentally the right way by understanding the following concepts.

## Believe that Long-Term Weight Loss is Possible through Intermittent Fasting

The first thing that you need to wrap your mind around is possibility. This is important because a lot of people are under the impression that there is this hot formula out there that they just need to adopt and things will be okay.

They're focusing more on things being okay, and the benefits they stand to get. I can't blame them for thinking this way, but here's the problem. You focus so much on the outcome that you run the risk of making the process unsustainable.

In other words, you're just looking at intermittent fasting as a process that produces the result that you want. You're focused more on the result kind of like the same way you desire a product.

However, here's the problem. If you do not fully believe in the process, you're making things much harder for yourself. In fact, if you don't believe it enough, weight loss is all but impossible. How come?

Well, you have your doubts. You're basically going through the motions. You're still unsure as to the feasibility of what you're doing. The bottom line if you have these beliefs, your heart wouldn't be in it. It's going to be very hard for you to commit. It's going to be very difficult for you.

## Practice Your Personal Focus with Mindfulness or Simple Stress Release

Weight loss is primarily a mental process. I know that sounds shocking because you probably have read so many diet books talking about the impact of food or certain supplements. You probably are a veteran of all sorts of weight loss physical exercise programs.

However, the truth is it's all in your head. It all boils down to your ability to focus. When you're focused, you are going to stick to doing something right here right now no matter how uncomfortable, inconvenient or downright painful it can be. You would be able to stick to doing the right even though it's very tempting to just flop down on your couch and play video games all day while eating a lot of fatty foods like potato chips.

You have to pay attention to your ability to focus. This is one key raw ingredient you have to be aware of. Once you understand that you need to focus, enhance your personal focus and powers. How? Practice mindfulness.

I'm not going to step you through the different flavors of mindfulness available to you. You can easily research this through Google. There is no shortage of mindfulness guides, booklets and cheat sheets available online. There are also complete books on this topic available on Amazon.

Regardless of the particular mindfulness method you use, you need to adopt some sort of mindfulness practice. When you're practicing mindfulness, you train your mind to stay on the ball. It doesn't stray. It doesn't get confused. It doesn't get distracted.

Instead, you train it to focus on one key element in the present moment. You're not worried about things that you think will happen in the future. You're not scared of what may possibly take place.

You're also not obsessing about mistakes from the past or traumatic experiences that happened. Think about it. They already happened. There's really nothing you can do about them. Kicking them around continuously in your mind is not doing anybody any favors.

When you practice mindfulness, you are able to, for lack of a better word, "unclench" your mind. You're not all caught up in the past, you're not worrying about the present nor are you distracted by what could possibly happen in the future.

Instead, you are at peace with one key stimulus that you're focusing on in the here and now. If you keep up, you will be able to conjure or call up that sense of inner calm so you can maximize your focus.

This is a very important skill because it enables you to do the right thing at the right time. When you adopt intermittent fasting, it's going to be tempting to eat outside the window. It's going to be tempting to change your sleeping schedule.

If you adopt a mindfulness practice and end up increasing your personal focusing abilities that way, you would be able to say no consistently. You would be able to tame yourself.

If this is too much of a leap of how you currently mentally operate, you can start things off low and slow. How? Practice simple stress release.

Navy Seals use a simple breathing technique that has been clinically proven to decrease stress by a lot. How simple is this technique?

Well, you only need to breathe in slowly and hold your breath for ten seconds. Slowly breathe out until there's no longer any air in your lungs and then hold it for ten seconds. Slowly breathe in again and repeat the process over and over. After about five repetitions, you will be very, very calm.

This works for most people. It doesn't matter how stressed you are. It doesn't matter how much trauma you're dealing with. This works for most people.

You probably would need to tweak the ten-second hold period. Maybe you can dial it down to four seconds if it's too much of a hassle. Whatever the case may be start with simple stress release. Once you're able to do that, try focusing and then once this has become second nature to you, adopt a mindfulness practice.

Again, there are many flavors of mindfulness out there. There's a lot to choose from.

## Be Clear on What Commitment is

Now that you have sharpened your personal focusing abilities, the next step is to be clear on what commitment is. Before you begin your intermittent fasting protocol, be clear that you are committing to it.

What is commitment? What does it require of you? You have to ask yourself what commitment is. This is a great way of reminding yourself.

Unfortunately, a lot of people do not take the time to stop and give themselves a reminder regarding commitment. They automatically assume that they can commit, and this is a big part of the problem.

When you remind yourself the definition of commitment, you are calling yourself out. You are asking yourself whether you have the ability to do this and whether you want it bad enough.

By doing this, you adopt an intermittent fasting protocol in a clear and intentional way. You don't just stumble into it. You don't just plunge into it headlong. Instead, it is something purposeful and deliberate.

Be clear on what commitment is and ask yourself are you ready to do this? Are you ready to go all the way?

**Commit to Starting**

Now that you're clear about what commitment is, you have to commit to a particular start date. This is a little tricky. Some people pick start dates that are very,

very imminent. These are start dates that are basically only a few days away. Others prefer a more distant start date like we're talking weeks, if not months.

Both of these are problematic. If you choose a start date that is too imminent, you might end up freaking yourself out. No joke. You might think that this is so close that you really have had no time to prepare. You end up intimidating yourself and making things harder on yourself. By the time the date comes, you find yourself completely unprepared.

The other extreme, of course, is setting up the start date too far ahead in the future. Here's the problem with that. As the old saying goes, "Life is what happens when you're making other plans".

Sure, you may have planned that you're going to start a month from now, but what do you think will happen to your life one month out? Well, this should not be a mystery. You will have other things to worry about. You will easily find other things to focus on.

What do you think happens when the start date comes? That's right. It will shock and surprise you. You will be as unprepared for this start date as you would be if you set it up ridiculously soon. Do you see how this works?

Do yourself a big favor and pick a start date that this neither too imminent nor too remote. This way you can plan ahead. This way you can commit to starting on time. It doesn't overcome you. It doesn't feel like a surprise. It definitely has a less of a chance of stressing you out.

## Take Baby Steps

When the start date comes for your intermittent fasting journey, take baby steps. In other words, don't worry about sticking to the schedule religiously from the get go. Maybe you were able to manage eating two hours outside the window. That's okay. It's much better than what you're doing now.

Chances are if you're struggling with your weight, you're probably eating a couple of meals in the morning, a couple of meals during the middle of the day and possibly a couple of meals late into the night. That's perfectly normal. A lot of people have that eating schedule.

When you allow yourself to take baby steps with your intermittent fasting protocol, you probably ate a meal a couple of hours or several hours outside the window. This is in stark contrast to how you normally eat. This, believe it or not, is a victory. Allow yourself to savor that victory.

It's okay to take baby steps. It's much better than what you had before. Most importantly, baby steps forward are still steps forward. They may seem small, they may seem insignificant but they're still important.

## Stick to Each Step

No matter how small the improvement is, allow yourself to understand what's going on. Allow yourself to see its importance. You have to understand that each step, no matter how small, is still a step in the right direction.

It's okay if you ate a couple of hours outside the window. It's okay if you overate within the window. That's fine. As long as you are narrowing the window, you are making progress. As long as you are getting used to the fact that you are doing this, you are making progress.

## Scale Up Over Time

The big challenge with scaling up has less to do with whether you should scale up or not. Believe it or not if you stick to a certain routine, it becomes second nature to you. It doesn't feel like some sort of hassle. It doesn't feel like some sort of heavy burden.

Again, once it becomes routine, it becomes easier and easier to stick to. You don't feel threatened by it. It doesn't feel like it hit you from left field. In fact, if you stick to it long enough, it feels like part of who you are. It seems so natural. This is precisely the point where you should consider scaling up.

Personally, I use this rule of thumb. Regardless of what I'm doing, maybe I'm doing weights, I'm doing fasting, I'm sticking to certain high-fat low-carb foods, I scale up when it has gotten easy.

For example, you are able to easily stick to eating within an eight-hour period out of every twenty-four-hour day. Maybe you add that eight-hour period right after you wake up or before you sleep. Regardless of how you do it, it's gotten easy. It's like second nature. That's when you should scale up because it doesn't feel like a chore to scale up.

You know you're in trouble when you're having a tough time eating within that time frame and now you're thinking of taking things to the next level and adopting Eat Stop Eat or eating only for four hours. That's not going to happen. I'm sorry to break it to you. Why? You're already having a tough time with 8-16 or 10-14. Can you imagine going with 4-20?

Pay attention to your mindset. Be honest whether it has gotten easy or you feel you're putting a lot of pressure on yourself. Again, it's okay to take baby steps. As long as you stick to each step, you will be okay.

## Develop a Daily Routine You Won't Deviate From

To make intermittent fasting a personal habit, you have to pair it with a set of signals that you routinely get every single day. In other words, you have to make it a routine. For example, if you work out in the morning, time your food intake from that point in time. This way when you turn your morning workouts into a habit, your intermittent fasting protocol automatically flows from it.

Usually, people are able to stick to a morning workout habit when they set up a trigger for themselves. Maybe it's an alarm clock. Perhaps it's a certain amount of light peering through their window. Whatever the case may be there is some sort of external trigger that reminds them to take habitual action.

Whatever the case may be, develop a daily routine that you won't deviate from. In fact in a 2009 study conducted by Jack F. Hollis with the Center for Health Research at Kaiser Permanente Northwest, effective weight loss boils down to the consistency of one's routine.

As long as you are consistent, you will achieve long-term weight loss. You won't be able to do this unless you develop a daily routine that you won't deviate from.

Remember intermittent fasting is just a tool. It's part of a larger context of lifestyle change so you have to shift into a different lifestyle.

# Chapter 5: Intermittent Fasting Protocols

As I mentioned in the previous chapter, intermittent fasting is actually straightforward. It's downright simple. It may not be easy but it's simple. It's all about reducing your eating window within a 24 hour day. This means that you are going to be extending the period within a 24 hour day that you are not eating. This sounds difficult.

To a lot of people, this is downright impossible. But they forget or overlook the fact that they're already fasting. I know it's kind of a shock, right? You probably don't think that you're in fasting but you are. Technically speaking, fasting is an extended period of time when you are not eating. That's the technical nutshell of fasting.

Can you find a time within a 24 hour period that you're doing that? This is the eye-opener. You're already doing it. It's called sleep. If you have a normal sleep pattern, you are fasting for at least eight hours a day. Intermittent fasting simply means that you're going to add additional hours to that eight hour period.

The amount of time you add depends on your gender. For men, it is recommended to fast for 16 hours and eat for eight hours. For women, the split is different. It is recommended that you fast for 14 hours and give yourself an eating window that spans 10 hours. Whatever the case may be, you are going to be splitting your time.

There are two ways to do it. You can add hours after you wake up or you can add the fasting hours before you go to bed. Those are your two broad options. Still, it's worth it to reiterate. You are already fasting. Get the idea out of your head that you're going to be doing something completely unheard of or strange. No, you're not. You're already doing this. It's called sleeping.

Unless you have some sort of weird sleepwalking habit where you eat while you sleep, you are fasting when you're sleeping. You're already doing this. The only thing left to do is to add time to your eight-hour sleeping window. This can be an additional eight hours or an additional six hours. It's also important to pick how you're going to do this.

Some people prefer the morning. So they basically give themselves until 10:00 AM to eat. Once they pass 10:00 AM, they stop eating. Alternatively, if you prefer dinners, you can give yourself until a certain time at night to eat. Whatever the case may be, it all boils down to adding hours to the amount of time you are already sleeping.

According to a 2018 study conducted by researcher Krista Varady of the University of Illinois, intermittent fasting using a 16/8 protocol is just as effective for losing weight as traditional diet. This means that for 16 hours, you're not eating and then eight hours you're eating. Varady and her team found that this can produce similar weight loss as traditional diets.

Now, you may be thinking that there's nothing to write about but you have to understand that intermittent fasting is not a diet. Yet it still produces similar results. Intermittent fasting, after all, is just scheduling your diet. This study was published in The Journal of Nutrition and Healthy Aging.

In another study released in 2016 by a team led by Michelle and Harvey from the University of Hospital of South Manchester LHS. Test animals were fed using an intermittent fasting schedule. Among the benefits observed by the team is the prolonged life and reduction of certain cancer risks. Keep in mind that this is on top of the weight loss these animals enjoyed. This is a 2016 study.

In another study in 2005, there was a link discovered between better blood sugar regulation and intermittent fasting. The study was conducted by Heilbronn LK with the Pennington Biomedical Research Center out of Baton Rouge, Louisiana. This study was originally published in the American Journal of Clinical Nutrition. As you can tell from these formal scientific peer-reviewed studies, intermittent fasting not only works but has a lot going for it in terms of health benefits.

# Chapter 6 : Getting Ready To Start

Now that you have a clear idea of what intermittent fasting is and you decided to get your head in the right place. As far as your assumptions and expectations are, it is time to get ready to start. This is your last checklist before you start your intermittent fasting protocol. You'll have to go through these and implement them. Don't skip a step.

## Put Together a Meal Plan for Your Eating Window

It's really important to break into intermittent fasting with a plan. Don't think that you're just going to continue doing what you're doing and do things by the seat of your pants. Don't expect to play it by ear. Why? The temptation to eat out of the window will probably get the better of you. It's only a matter of time.

It may not happen immediately but it can and will catch up to you. You might not do it right out of the gate but if you think you can just do things based on what you feel like, you're really making things harder on yourself. You're not doing yourself any favors. Stick to a plan at least for the first couple of weeks. It doesn't have to be elaborate.

It doesn't have to break everything down in terms of calorie count and whether you've covered all the major food groups. There's no need to do that. There's no need to slice and dice your meal plan. Just have a plan. In fact, the simpler it is, the more likely you will stick to it. Put that meal plan together. The question that is begging to be asked of course is what you are going to put in your plan. What kind of foods should you focus on? Here are some guidelines:

**Focus on Taste**

You should know enough about yourself to identify your taste preference. Some people prefer salty foods. Other people prefer sweets. Whatever the case may be, identify your taste profile and stick to it. Focus on taste. When you're putting together your meal plan, load up on the stuff that you think that tastes good. I wish I could tell you that there's some sort of one size fits all answer. There isn't. Everybody has different taste preferences. Just focus on what you like. Focus on what's delicious.

## Focus on Satiety

Now that you're putting together your meal plan in terms of taste, you have to add another layer. Now that you know that you prefer certain foods that taste a certain way. Maybe you like salty and fatty foods. Identify the foods that fit their distaste profile in terms of how likely they are to fill you up.

Again, if you've been eating a lot of foods that fall within a certain flavor range, this should be quite apparent that you should be able to identify these hoots. Knowing what you know and based on your eating patterns, focus on the foods that fill you up and keep you feeling full for the longest time. This is the key to satiety. It's not enough that these dishes taste great. That's great and everything but you're adding an extra consideration.

You're looking to eat only foods that not only taste good but keep you feeling full for much longer. When you list down all the foods that you normally eat, it should be fairly clear which dishes keep you full for a far longer period of time.

## Rotate These Dishes So You Don't Get Bored Out Of Your Routine

One of the most common complaints about most diets and weight loss programs is that they get boring really quickly. Take the case of the Atkins diet. A lot of people who adopt that diet end up eating only a narrow range of food. In the first few weeks, they do really well. They lose a lot of fat. They're feeling good about their weight loss.

But sooner or later, they hit a wall. Given enough time, they drop the diet. What happened? Their meal plans got boring. They just stuck to the same foods. It's as if they're using some sort of formula. They keep going through the formula over and over until it got boring.

Don't let this happen to you. You have to rotate the dishes based on the analytical steps above in such a way that you don't get bored. When you get bored, it's so easy to drop your routine. It's so easy to just basically go back to your own eating habits. That's not going to work. You have to understand that this can be an issue. So you have to get enough meal ideas together and schedule them in such a way that they do not get boring.

In a 2015 study led by psychologist Lucy Chambers from the University of Sussex, high protein and high fiber foods were shown to aid weight loss significantly. People who included such items on their meal plans made people felt fuller for a longer period of time. Focus on satiety when making meal plan decisions.

It's not enough to go with dishes that you know taste great. Eating delicious food is one thing. Eating delicious food that makes you feel fuller for a longer period of time so you reduce your calorie intake is another thing entirely. Know the difference.

# Chapter 7 : Induction Period

The intermittent fasting's induction period is the point when you just start the I.F. Protocol. This period gets your system ready. You basically switch to a new lifestyle. This can also be very stressful. Like it or not. It can be very challenging. After all, you're going from a lifestyle where you're not really paying attention to when you eat to one where eating schedules are extremely important.

Don't expect the transition to be smooth. This is also the most common mistakes people make. They think that since intermittent fasting is all about scheduling eating then it necessarily follows that they can just jump into it. I wish it were that easy. Because if you think that it was going to be easy and you end up stumbling when you start, it's too tempting to conclude that you've failed.

When you reach that conclusion, it's easy to take things to the next level and use this as an excuse to stop. Do you see how this works? Like I mentioned in the previous chapter, your mind and your body are going to be playing tricks on you. You're basically going to end up trying to sabotage yourself. Remember we're all creatures of habit.

We grow accustomed to doing things a certain way and unless we are mindful of how our systems respond to the lifestyle choices we end up falling back to our old routines. Be aware that there is an induction period and that you have to make proper changes to your lifestyle.

Work on getting full sleep. The first thing that you need to do to snap into or fall into an intermittent fasting protocol and eating schedule is to get enough sleep. Now, there is no formula for this. The conventional wisdom is you should get eight hours of sleep.

Actually many people do well with seven hours. Some people even do fine with six hours. Whatever the case may be, pay attention to how well you feel when you sleep eight hours, seven hours, or six hours. Don't push it. For example, if you sleep for eight hours and you feel groggy when you wake up then this should be the cue that you slept too long.

Just focus on your energy level and your mental clarity. However, your body defines the term "a full night's sleep" stick to it. Again, this could be anywhere from six to eight hours. Some people prefer nine hours. Regardless, work on getting full sleep. You should be able to transition into this after a few days or maybe a week or two.

## Eat a Big Breakfast or Dinner

At this point, you're going to decide how you're going to put together your intermittent fasting window. Are you going to add to the hours you slept or are you going to add to the hours you slept before you wake up, before you sleep, or after you sleep? This is a big decision because this is going to lead to you either eating a big breakfast or a big dinner meal.

Whatever the case may be, focus on what feels right and natural to you. Stick with what seems easy as far as your eating preferences are concerned. Try not to buck your body system. Just add an early meal or just focus on an early meal or a late meal.

## Focus on Getting Used To Your Big Meals within the Time Period

One of the most common rookie mistakes people make when adopting an intermittent fasting eating schedule is to assume that they really have all the time in the world to eat a meal. It then dawns on them that they have to cut off all meals past a certain time. For example, if you prefer to eat in the morning, a good cutoff point would be 4:00 in the afternoon or earlier.

For example, if you wake up at 6:00 in the morning, it's a good idea to prefer the morning for your intermittent fasting eating window. It's a good idea to stop eating past 2:00 o'clock. Regardless of how you schedule it when you first start your intermittent fasting journey, it's easy to forget this. So you're thinking to yourself of all the time in the world to eat. Basically, you're thinking about your regular eating schedule.

So what happens? You might make a mistake and you eat outside the window. This is why it's a good idea to get your big meals out of the way first. In other words, have a big breakfast or have a big dinner. When you do this, you concentrate satiety into that timeframe and sooner or later you start equating or associating being full with a specific meal. It could be a dinner. It could be lunch. It could be breakfast.

## Don't Feel Too Bad If You Eat Outside the Window

Believe me. I understand what you're going through right now. Right now, you're really pumped up. You're really committed to sticking within the window. You were saying to yourself I'm going to do this. I'm going to eat within my intermittent fasting window. Congratulations. Good job. Good job on committing.

Here's the problem though. Since this is the induction period and you're really just going to ease into this. Don't expect things to be smooth. You have to understand that you are a creature of your habits. You've grown accustomed to doing things a certain way. You're still have not completely transformed your lifestyle.

Right now, you're just operating based solely on the idea of intermittent fasting. You're thinking that it would be a good thing to switch to this schedule. You understand the benefits it brings to the table. That's all well and good but thinking about doing things is one thing.

Actually doing them is another thing entirely. I say this because you should not feel too bad if you eat outside the window. It's not the end of the world. You did not break your promise to yourself. You did not fail. The problem a lot of people have with commitment is that they often think that if they break their commitment, it's game over.

They've broken their word to themselves. All bets are off. What we are really doing when we look at the situation in black and white terms like this is we are giving ourselves an excuse to fail all the way. Don't play that game with yourself. Just understand that you made a mistake and that's fine. You're still doing well.

Why? Compare this to how you ate before. Right now, you may have eaten two hours outside your window. This is bad but it's not even close to what you were doing before. You would eat throughout the day except for the eight hours or so that you are sleeping. I mean how many calories do you think you were packing in when you were eating like that.

Don't make things hard on yourself by being an absolutist. Understand that this is still progress. Sure if you ate outside the window. But this is not the end of the world. You're getting closer. Look at this as an important step forward. It may be a small step but it's still a step forward.

## Keep Focusing on Eating within the Window until you're Able to Stick to It

Focus on your schedule when can you start eating and when do you have to stop eating. Again, don't beat yourself up if you eat outside the window. But the more you focus on it, the more you hold yourself accountable. You now have a metric. You now have some sort of benchmark.

This enables you to come back to the benchmark again and again until you get closer and closer to the window. Eventually, you would reach a point where you're just eating within the window. For some people, this is fairly easy and straightforward. For the rest of us, it can be quite a challenge. The key is to just focus on that window.

Don't focus on the fact that you ate outside the window. Don't think that this is the end of the world. Just focus on the window. You know where it is. Sure you ate outside of it but it's okay because you know where it is. You know where to go back to. So the next time you slip up, you get closer and closer to the window. Eventually, you reach a point where you get so used to the window that you eat within it. You will be able to stick to it.

# Chapter 8: Turbo Charge Weight Loss with the Right Yummy Food

By this point, you should've started your intermittent fasting protocol. You should've gone through the induction period by eating the stuff that you normally eat.

The key here is to direct your attention to stuff that either contains more fiber or fat. When you do that, you feel fuller for a longer period of time.

Also, since you're eating food that fits your taste preferences, you are less likely to fall off the wagon. Why? Well, you're eating stuff that you like. You're eating stuff that tastes good to you. This tricks your system into thinking that you're really not doing anything out of the ordinary.

The only different thing that you're doing is that you're choosing to eat either a little bit earlier, or a little bit later than normal. You're also choosing to eat within a specific time frame. That's it. That's all that's changed.

Again, since you are being flexible about this and not beating yourself up if you eat outside of your eating window, this process should be a fairly smooth one for you. Stick to this for quite some time.

Keep at it until you get used to it. In the beginning you'd probably be eating a few hours outside your target window, but as you get used to your new eating schedule, you'll be able to stick to this window more closely.

Maybe you'd start out three hours out. Then, after a week, you'd be able to get it down to two hours out. After that, it's one hour out. After a whole month, you'll be within your window and after another month, you'll get closer to the beginning of that window.

In other words, you'll start mastering your eating schedule. Once you become comfortable with your schedule, level up. That's right. This is the time to scale up. How?

Turbo charge your weight loss by eating the right yummy food. In other words, focus on high fat foods. You have to understand that our ancestors thousands of years ago preferred fatty foods. In fact, according to some research studies, that's what they ate primarily.

It's easy to see why. When you eat fatty foods, you feel fuller for a longer period of time. You also get maximum return for the food that you eat. You can eat less food which packs so much calories and energy that you'll still have the energy you need to get on with the rest of your day.

This is why with everything else being equal, our ancestors preferred fatty food. That worked back then. It will work right here, right now.

Add high fat foods to your meal plan. Again, this is the key. Displace. Do not replace. Don't interpret this as an instruction for you to clear stuff off your plate to make room for high-fat, low-carb foods.

No. If you're doing that, you're doing it wrong. Just add on to your current meal plan. The key is to focus on foods that satisfy you richly and quickly. These foods hit you with a punch. You know you fill full and that you've had enough. This lasts a longer time.

If you do this correctly, you'll end up displacing stuff that you normally eat like bread, sugary snacks, or stuff that you eat throughout the day. They're not as filling. They're not as satisfying. They don't pack as much of a punch.

Again, this doesn't happen overnight. Allow the displacement process to work itself out.

**Get used to high-fat foods**

It's important that you are completely mindful of your personal flavor preferences. It doesn't really matter whether you're into salty foods, sour foods, or whatnot. There will always be a fatty variation of that food.

Focus on the flavor, but load up on the fat. Keep this up for quite some time. Sooner or later, you're going to have to make a fairly difficult move.

A lot of people have a tough time with this next step. I can't say I can blame them. It's easy to get hooked on sugar. There are a lot of people who are truly sugar addicts.

The key here is to start ramping down on carbs. I keep saying this, but it's absolutely true. This is not going to happen overnight. Give yourself some time.

As long as you're staying within your window, you are in a good spot. Get ready to cut down on carbs. Load up on fat. Get used to them. Then, start cutting down on the pasta, rice, potatoes, and noodles. Definitely cut out soda drinks.

The secret

What is the secret to finally kicking the carb habit? Believe me, it is a habit. Well, stick to staying within your eating window for 21 days and eat more and more fat, and less and less carbs.

If you do this for 21 days and you're able to stick to it, it becomes a habit. You start seeking high-fat, low-carb foods. Most importantly, you eat all of these within your eating window.

Just how important is cutting carbs out of your diet? Just how much of a weight loss impact does cutting carbs out of your diet have? According to a 2011 Harvard University study led by Dariush Mozaffarian, people who changed their intake of sugars, fats, refined grains, and other foods high in starch had the most weight change.

In other words, if you are looking to change your weight one way or the other, you should start looking at those foods. Either you eat more of them if you're underweight, or you eat less of them if you're overweight.

Similarly, there was also a 2010 study published in the New England Journal of Medicine which was conducted by Thomas Meinert. The study says that increasing a diet's protein content and reducing carb levels enables people to keep whatever weight they lost through diets off.

Finally, in a 2012 cross study review involving 50 diet studies, a team out of the University of Helsinki, Finland, led by Mikael Fogelholm, found that the more carbs and sugar one eats, the fatter one gets over a period of time. All these studies highlight the importance of modifying and eventually, cutting back on carb levels, as far as food choices go.

# Chapter 9 : Intermittent Fasting Turbocharges Ketogenic Weight Loss

By this point, your mind should be open to a high-fat, low-carb diet. Maybe it will take you a few months to get here. Maybe it will take you close to a year. Whatever the case may be, if you followed all the steps that I've outlined previously in this book, you will get to this point.

Now, you may be thinking, "I understand that you want me to load up on fat and reduce carbs while eating a moderate level of protein, but what is the upside? How does this work in general? What should I look forward to?"

Well, please understand that when you adopt a high-fat, low-carb diet, not only do you feel fuller for longer periods of time which leads to sustained weight loss, you also turbo charge your body's ability to burn fat. I know it sounds paradoxical, but it's true.

To burn fat more efficiently, you have to eat more fat. If you think about it from a metabolic perspective, this makes all the sense in the world. If you're eating a lot of carbs, the carbs in your system triggers insulin production.

Whenever insulin makes an appearance in your bloodstream, it shuts down your cells' ability to burn fat as fuel. If this isn't bad enough, the insulin presence in your bloodstream also seals off your cells from releasing fat compounds for energy. This is a double whammy.

If you eat too much sugar, you develop insulin resistance. You have to eat more and more sugar to trigger your body's insulin response. This leaves more and more sugar in your bloodstream.

Sugar is actually toxic. Until and unless your cells absorb and burn them for energy, when left in your bloodstream, they act like little knives that cut up your system and inflame your tissues. Bad news.

In fact, insulin spikes are the reason why people who eat high-carb diets eat throughout the day. They are hungry throughout the day.

## Add and Displace, Not Replace

Please understand that if you want to adopt a ketogenic diet, you have to use a displacement strategy. Eat more cream cheese, eggs, butter, and avocados.

Once your taste change to these, you'll find it easier to skip out on starchy foods like potatoes, pasta, rice, and others. Your taste will also change and shift from donuts, cakes, and cookies to fatty foods.

## Quick Warning Regarding Protein

One of the easiest ways that people who are looking to adopt a ketogenic use to make the switch is to eat more protein. They're thinking that when they do this, they automatically load up on fat.

This is not necessarily the case. For example, if you are going to be eating chicken breast, that is one of the leanest parts of the chicken especially when the skin is taken off. In fact, the moment you take off chicken skin, you're pretty much eating lean meat because the skin is where the chicken stores most of its fat.

Do not adopt a high-protein diet and assume that it' is a high-fat diet. These are two totally different things. On a high-fat, low-carb diet, you are using fat as your main energy source.

You have minimal levels of insulin so this means your body is primed to burn fat compounds called ketones as its primary source of energy. With less insulin, you're also priming your cells to release fat regularly for processing by your liver.

You get more ketones. You burn the ketones and you get thinner and thinner because you're burning through your fat layer.

You can easily short-circuit this beautiful process by loading up on protein. Why? Chemically speaking, your liver can turn protein into glucose, also known as sugar.

When this happens, insulin enters the picture and your struggle with fat burning resumes again. I'm not saying that you should cut out protein all together. You just need to reduce it to a moderate level.

If you are eating 70% fat, try not to eat more than 20% protein and 10% carbs. Regardless of what you do, the total amount of carbs you eat every single day once you have fully transitioned to a high-fat, low-carb diet should be no more than 12 grams.

I know. This seems like a tall order, but like I said, if you transition to this stage, this will turn out to be much easier than you originally anticipated.

Just how much of a role does sugar play in weight gain and weight retention?

In 2013, there was a study from University of Otago which was published by Lisa Te Morenga. Her team's analysis of 68 different studies indicate that the more people ate sugar, the more they struggled with their weight. This has something to do with insulin control.

In fact, in a 2018 study out of Chungnam National University in South Korea led by E Cha, the research team found that stabilizing blood sugar levels led to better health outcomes. This included weight loss, as well as avoiding certain types of chronic diseases.

Finally, in a 2013 study, fat metabolism specialist Ellen Blaak from Maastricht University discovered that there is a tight link between obesity and blood sugar levels. The study says that poor control of blood sugar leads to obesity as well as heart diseases and Type 2 Diabetes. This is due to the role insulin plays in metabolism.

Taken as a whole, all these three studies reiterate the role that insulin and blood sugar levels play in fat metabolism and overall weight loss.

# Chapter 10: Get Ready to Scale Up

By this point, you should have adopted a ketogenic diet. Things are probably going smoothly for you because you've been able to stick to your new eating lifestyle for more than 21 days.

Congratulations. It has become a habit. It is no longer some sort of fluke or some phase that you're going through. This is real. Pat yourself in the back.

If you did stick to it, a lot of that weight that you have lost are not going to come back anytime soon. With that said, if things have become easier for you and if things have become routine, you might want to take things to the next level.

You may be thinking that you've already taken things to the next level by adopting a ketogenic diet. That's all well and good, but if you really want to maximize the power of intermittent fasting, it's time to emphasize the fasting portion of the phrase "intermittent fasting".

In other words, you're going to extend the no-eating period way outside of that 8-16 or 10-14 eating window. You're going to level up to the point where you're actually going to go a full day without eating. Here's how you do it.

**Eat-Stop-Eat**

Eat-stop-eat, as the name indicates, simply means that you're going to eat for one day and then, stop and then, eat for another day. The secret to this is to transition from your tight window discipline of 8-16 or 10-14 to 24-8-24.

In other words, you're going to divide the calendar in such a way that you're going to do fasting for 24 hours straight. It may seem like a harsh transition, but if you reached this stage where things are very easy for you, this is not as hard as you think.

In fact, if you have reached a point where you actually eat only once a day or you eat within a tiny window like a one-hour or 30-minute window every day, adopting an eat-stop-eat schedule by simply stretching out the timelines won't seem like any change in your lifestyle. Seriously.

Think about it. If you have become so disciplined as to eat only within an hour every single day and have a good time the rest of the day, you can reach a point where you make that hour shrink down to 30 minutes and then later on, to 15 minutes.

Past that point when you have easily made that transition, it's not all that hard to make that 15 minutes disappear altogether. You'll end up fasting for a 24-hour period. This is how you transition into an eat-stop-eat protocol.

Unfortunately, a lot of people jump straight to eat-stop-eat. They don't even take the time to master intermittent fasting.

I'm sorry to report that most of these people end up failing. It's just too hard on their system. They can't quite make the transition.

Now, don't get me wrong. I'm not saying that they don't succeed initially. In fact, a lot of them are able to do this for months, but eventually, their old lifestyle habits and eating patterns catch up to them and they end up where they began.

It's much better to master intermittent fasting. Reduce your eating window to a few hours, and then an hour, and then a few minutes, until you can smoothly switch to 24-hour no-eating periods.

## 3-2-3

When you switch to a 3-2-3 protocol, you eat within a tiny window for three days straight. Basically, you just practice intermittent fasting the way you've been practicing them.

You do this for three days straight. Then, you transition to two days of absolutely no eating. After that, you go back to your three-day schedule.

This might seem like quite a bit of an abrupt change, but if you smoothly transition to eat-stop-eat, 3-2-3 is not that hard. It's not going to be that difficult.

The key here is to scale up once things seem normal. Once you think that sticking to your schedule has become easy and part of your routine, that's when you level up. The 3-2-3 schedule is the next natural stage after you've mastered eat-stop-eat.

## 3-4-3

If you have mastered 3-2-3, the next step is to go with 3-4-3. I'm not going to go past this because anything after this would be too disruptive.

You'd probably be able to stick to longer fasts, but that's not the issue. The problem is, eventually, this will catch up to you. Maybe schedule changes. Maybe there are all sorts of pressure or stresses in your life.

Personally speaking, 3-4-3 was the best I was able to manage. I was able to do this given the normal pressures and stresses of my life. Since this book is based on my personal experience, this is the best I can recommend.

You can lose quite a bit of weight with the 3-4-3 protocol because you're going without food for four days straight. Think about that, 96 hours without food. That's a lot of calorie burning. That's a lot of fat metabolization.

Pat yourself on the back if you're able to stick to that. After that, you just need to maintain a 3-4-3 distribution.

# Conclusion

Make no mistake. If you want to lose weight, you need to adopt a new routine. There are many fad diets out there. The reason why they've become fads in the first place is they work at some level or other.

Let me tell you, Diet Book is not going to become a best seller if it does not work. People who've tried it and strictly implemented the steps ended up losing weight. That's not the problem here.

The issue is how long that weight will stay off. This is where most diets fall apart. They can teach you how to lose weight, but they cannot teach you how to become disciplined. They cannot teach you how to incorporate these weight loss protocols into your daily routine.

In other words, these weight loss techniques remain techniques that are outside of you. They're just things that you try on from time to time or for a certain period of time and then, you try something else. This is why most people fail with long-term weight loss.

You don't have to be another statistic. By adopting intermittent fasting, you make certain changes to your lifestyle which changes your attitude, mindset, and expectations. These lead to profound and sustainable weight loss. I wish you nothing but the very best weight loss success.

## DISCLAIMER

While all attempts have been made to verify the information provided in this publication, the author does not assume any responsibility for errors, omissions, or contrary interpretations of the subject matter herein.

The views expressed are those of the author alone and should not be taken as expert instruction or commands. The reader is responsible for his or her own actions.

The author makes no representations or warranties with respect to the accuracy or completeness of the contents of this work and specifically disclaims all warranties, including without limitation warranties of fitness for a particular purpose. No warranty may be created or extended by sales or promotional materials. The advice and recipes contained herein may not be suitable for everyone. This work is sold with the understanding that the author is not engaged in rendering medical, legal or other professional advice or services. If professional assistance is required, the services of a competent professional person should be sought. The author shall not be liable for damages arising here from. The fact that an individual, organization of website is referred to in this work as a citation and/or potential source of further information does not mean that the author endorses the information the individual, organization to website may provide or recommendations they/it may make. Further, readers should be aware that Internet websites listed in this work might have changed or disappeared between when this work was written and when it is read.

Adherence to all applicable laws and regulations, including international, federal, state, and local governing professional licensing, business practices, advertising, and all other aspects of doing business in any jurisdiction in the world is the sole responsibility of the purchaser or reader.

Made in the USA
Lexington, KY
24 September 2018